D1539208

How To Do
Restorative Yoga
For Home or in a Class

by Michael Hetherington
(L.Ac & Yoga Teacher)

Disclaimer

All material in this book is provided for your information only and may not be construed as medical advice or instruction. No action or inaction should be taken based solely on the contents of this information; instead, readers should consult appropriate health professionals on any matter relating to their health and well-being.

The information and opinions expressed here are believed to be accurate, based on the best judgment available to the authors, and readers who fail to consult with appropriate health authorities assume the risk of any injuries. The publisher is not responsible for errors or omissions.

About the Author

Michael Hetherington is a qualified acupuncturist, health practitioner and yoga teacher based in Brisbane, Australia. He has a keen interest in mind-body medicine, energetic anatomy, yoga nidra and Buddhist style meditation. Inspired by the teachings of many he has learned that a light-hearted, joyful approach to life serves best.

Other Titles by Author:

Chakra Balancing Made Simple and Easy

The Complete Book of Oriental Yoga

Meditation Made Simple

The Little Book of Yin

How to Learn Acupuncture

Simply Zen Quotes

Acknowledgements

I would like to thank the Peter Masters and the other teachers at Zen Central Yoga Studio in Brisbane, Australia for showing me the path of yoga in a playful and joyful way. I would also like to thank Angela for posing in the photos and providing many hours of insightful discussion. And thank you to all of the students, teachers and masters from the past that have helped to guide the way.

Table of Contents

Introduction

"Do your practice, all is coming." ~ Sri K Pattabhi Jois

Restorative yoga is a gentle form of yoga. It can be practiced by anyone, anytime, by beginners or advanced yoga practitioners. It serves to bring more flexibility, musculoskeletal and emotional release, and quietude of mind.

This simple book is to help outline the approach to restorative forms of yoga. I have provided some fundamental principles to act as a guide to help you practice in a safe and supportive manner. Please read all this information before starting the poses.

Many of the poses can be adapted to suit your level of mobility and the resources available. It is encouraged that you experiment with various poses once you become familiar with the main poses outlined in this book.

Deep kinesthetic awareness develops through the practice of gentle and restorative yoga. A developed kinesthetic awareness helps you to move your body in more effective and efficient ways. It also helps you to become more sensitive and attuned to various environments, to other people, and to your own inner intelligence and wisdom.

Within the scope of any yoga practice there are almost limitless postures and practices that one can explore. This is also true for restorative and other gentle forms of yoga. However, for the benefit of this book, I have chosen to simplify the practice to keep it uncomplicated, and therefore accessible to all levels and abilities. The postures outlined in this book are more than enough to either get you started on your journey, or provide you some extra insight into your already established yoga practice. If after reading and applying the lessons in this book you are ready to move on, then I encourage you to find a class and a teacher near you.

Why Restorative and Gentle Yoga?

More often than not, people are living very busy lives; they work hard, they play hard, and they exercise harder. There is a common idea in the West that we need to engage only in exercises that require great effort, and in some cases great pain, to receive any benefits. This is not the whole truth. Sometimes, a little stress can be helpful—it gets us going, it stresses the muscle tissues so that they can repair and rebuild stronger than before, and it provides us with a way to channel any excess energy. Yet, what is really lacking in our understanding is that we need both the "yin" and the "yang" to progress in any aspect of our lives. A lifestyle full of running around, working hard, playing hard and exercising harder is purely a "yang" pursuit. "Yin" is often overlooked and is sometimes viewed as boring, as it involves sitting quietly, taking time out, meditating, breathing slowly, resting, taking baths, and doing gentle exercise forms that focus on increasing internal awareness.

In any case, for the body and nervous system to adapt, learn, grow and develop, it needs some time to reorganize itself. It needs time out from all the "yang" style activities so it can reorganize and settle into a new pattern and a new way of being. That way, when it comes to "yang" time again, the body is ready and willing.

One of the ways you can actually drain your energies and cause harm to your body and mind is to overexert. This can come about from using an incorrect technique in which you are using more energy than is actually required to do a task, and/or it can come from simply doing too much too often, without enough rest. When the body and mind are given an adequate chance to rest and restore, you will find that when you return to the "yang" activity, you can actually perform that activity much better than before.

If we don't allow the body this time to rest and renew itself, you can simply compound the amount of stress in the body and mind until eventually something will give out—an injury, a midlife crisis, an anxiety attack, a torn ligament, a slipped disc, etc. All these incidences may be signs from our bodies and minds that we are overexerting ourselves, and therefore they are telling us that we need to find more balance in our lives. Simply put, we need to take regular time out for moments of self-inquiry, and engage in gentle practices that support the cultivation of internal awareness rather than chasing after external stimulation.

This is why practices like restorative and other gentle forms of yoga are needed in our lives. They give us the chance to reestablish balance and to support our "yang" activities, and they help to cultivate our inner selves.

These practices are also suitable for beginners who are looking to get into yoga, but who don't feel ready to attend the general classes being offered. This is a great place to start, because in this book we work gently, patiently and supportively. We can allow a deeper relationship with our body to take place so that when we feel ready to attend general classes, we have the fundamentals in place. It will also provide you with the advantage of having already established a relationship with your body; therefore, you will receive more benefit from general classes.

I encourage everyone to take more time out to practice these gentle forms of yoga alongside any other activities you are engaged in and see if, and how, restorative yoga helps to improve your performance in those other activities over time.

Please do not attempt poses with an attitude of "I have to" or "I must do this", as if it is a chore; rather, see it as an opportunity to take some time out and nurture yourself. Allow yourself to see it as a journey, where you can discover new sensations and spaces within yourself that you were previously unaware of. Knowing how to use this approach will also benefit the other elements of your life.

Relinquish the mind, be gentle with yourself and go within.

Enjoy the journey.

How to Use This Book

Firstly, read the "Fundamentals" chapter to help you establish a safe practice and a safe approach.

Next is a chapter dedicated purely to explaining the poses themselves, in no particular order.

Then, in the chapter titled "Practice Sequences", I have put these poses together in various orders, depending on the amount of time available, and whether there are any particular parts of the body that you are looking to work with more specifically.

After that chapter, I have provided you with a list of resources you can use if you want to develop your practice further, or if you are looking for yoga props and materials to support your practice.

Finally, for those who may be interested, I have put together a little chapter at the end to explain a little about my story, and how I came to write this book and to be attracted to this form of yoga.

So without further ado, let's learn how to do restorative yoga!

Fundamentals

Below is a list of fundamental principles to guide your practice. They are designed to keep you safe, avoid injury, and equip you with a gentle and supportive attitude. Please read them carefully and understand them before moving into practicing the poses.

A SAFE PRACTICE

Do not force anything; restorative yoga is done in a gentle and organic way. It takes time for some tissues in the body to respond to the pose, so just wait, find your breath, and progressively relax the body as you begin to "feel into it". If you force the body and joints where they don't want to go, your body will give you a number of signals:

1. The breath may become tight and you may tend to hold your breath
2. You may experience a sharp shooting pain
3. Something around the joint just won't feel right

When any of these happen, pull back! If you keep going, it is likely that you will have a muscle spasm, overstretch a ligament, or compromise the joint—and if any of these things happen, they will have you hobbling around for at least six weeks, unable to do much until your body recovers. It's not worth it! Be patient and gentle with yourself, and use your abilities of awareness to move your body with integrity.

AN OPEN AND CURIOUS MIND

MOVE INTO THE POSES SLOWLY AND GENTLY

A DEEPENED AND SENSITIVE AWARENESS OF YOUR INTERNAL ENVIRONEMNT is more important and more powerful than achieving, or looking like you have achieved any particular yoga pose.

USE SUPPORT PROPS WHEN REQUIRED (bolsters, pillows, blankets), especially around the joints (knees, hips, neck). The body has a natural defense system that is activated when it feels like the joints are under threat; the muscles in the area will seize up to protect the joint. This is what happens when you have a muscle spasm in the back for instance (the joint was under threat, so to avoid a serious injury, the muscles go into "freak-out mode" and seize up to protect the joint at all cost). So to avoid this situation, use support when required—then the joints won't feel so threatened, and the musculature will be able to relax and release.

PRACTICE IN A QUIET AND CLEAN ENVIRONMENT

PRACTICE ON A FIRM YET SOFT SURFACE THAT IS FLAT
The ideal surface would to be a futon on the floor. Next best after that would be a thick yoga mat on the floor. I like to bulk up the padding if I'm on the floor, so use blankets, rugs or carpeted areas if possible. If you use a blanket, keep it neat and folded when using it; don't let it scrunch up and unbalance things. You can practice some poses in your bed if you like, but because of the softness of the mattress and the different angles this creates, make sure you don't fall asleep in the poses or hold them for over five minutes.

YOUR BEST FRIEND IS YOUR BREATH
Keep coming back to it when the mind wanders for too long.

GIVE YOURSELF AT LEAST 10 MINTUES TO PRACTICE
You will probably get 2 – 4 poses done in that time. Ideally, especially in a class environment, the time of practice would be at least ninety minutes. It is great to practice at home, but **when you can, participate in a class.** Many people find it much easier to practice in a group environment. There is a collective focus of energy that is available in the class environment. It also gives you a chance to have some time and space away from your daily life, and gives you an opportunity to learn from a teacher who is most likely very experienced with that particular style of yoga. A good teacher provides a safe, supportive, informative and comfortable atmosphere to practice in.

IT IS NOT COMPETITIVE... LEAVE THE EGO AT THE DOOR

Materials Recommended

1. A soft yet firm surface that you can lie flat on. A thin futon is preferable but a thick yoga mat will also be suitable.

2. At least two blankets, and a few pillows

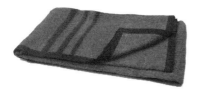

3. At least one yoga bolster. Yoga bolsters are perfect for this practice but not everyone has one—so be resourceful. Bolsters are chunky, so you will need to replace them with lots of pillows or cushions if you don't have one.

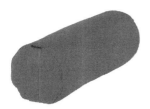

4. Warm things: warm clothes, socks, extra blankets, heaters if suitable. Warmth helps your blood and energy flow more easily through your body.

5. Nice music helps. Any ambient music, I find, works great. Slow hypnotic music, world music, maybe some classical.

6. Water and fluids. Warm water is best; avoid ice cold water (it's not good for your stomach). Cups of herbal tea close by would be picture perfect.

Check out the "Resources" chapter if you're looking for suppliers of these materials.

That's it! Ready, Set . . . . . . Slow down.

Breathe.

"Fear cannot enter a quiet heart."

~ Paramahansa Yogananda

The Poses Explained

"If a man insisted always on being serious, and never allowed himself a bit of fun and relaxation, he would go mad or become unstable without knowing it."

~ Herodotus

Butterfly Pose

1. Bring the soles of your feet together. Allow some space between the heels of your feet and your groin—no need to jam yourself up.

2. Grab your feet, or interlace your fingers around your toes (it doesn't really matter which); inhale to lengthen through your spine, exhale to draw yourself gently forward and down.

3. Take your time to soften into the pose. Connective tissue in the body takes at least thirty seconds to respond, so just go easy into it.

4. After thirty seconds to one minute, allow your back to curl and your head to soften towards the floor. Let gravity do the work! Relax your shoulders, arms, legs, and head, and sink towards the floor. Closing the eyes can be very powerful here. Stay for at least three minutes if comfortable.

5. For extra comfort and support, use a yoga bolster to rest your head on. When the body feels the support, it will naturally start to release and relax. Keep your breath smooth and gentle. Stay for at least three minutes if comfortable; if not comfortable and then come up whenever you're ready.

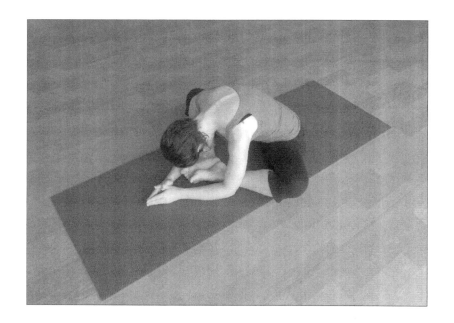

Supported Butterfly

1. Similar to the butterfly pose, the differences being that you bring in a bolster and some pillows in between the knees to rest your head on for extra support.

Variations:

1. If your knees are uncomfortably up, and/or your lower back is curling out and it's uncomfortable, then try sitting up on a few blankets to raise your hips away from the floor, and then try again.

2. If you find that you can't relax your legs and allow the knees to move towards the floor, then put some pillows underneath the knees and legs so they feel supported. If the knee joint feels threatened, the muscles will tighten up naturally to protect it. You will need to support the knee joint so that it feels supported; only then will it allow itself to let go.

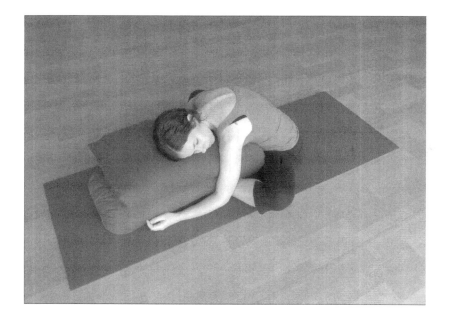

Massage the Legs

It's always a good idea to incorporate a little leg and foot massage into any restorative yoga practice.

The insides of your legs are the "yin" channels, and the outsides of your legs are the "yang" channels. For restorative and relaxation purposes, it is best to work with the feet and insides of the legs.

1. Start by accessing just one of your feet. Start to work the thumb pads into the inner arches of that foot. When you find tender points, hold the pressure; it should decrease in tenderness after a little while. Keep massaging the foot.

2. Start working the thumb pads into the underbelly of the foot. Again, if you come across tender points, give them more attention by holding a gentle pressure on them and letting the tenderness dissipate.

3. Allow your hands to work up to the inside of the ankle, and use you palm to squeeze the inside of the ankle. Be gentle yet firm.

4. Now, let the hands work up the insides of the lower leg, again using your palms to squeeze gently. I also use my thumbs to add pressure just under the shinbone, like in the picture below. Be gentle; the insides of the legs will generally be more tender and sensitive than the outsides of the legs.

5. Work your way all the way up to the knee, and give the knee a bit of a squish and massage. Feel free to adjust your leg so it is comfortable for you and for your knee.

6. When you feel like you've had enough, let that leg go and begin on the other foot and leg. Repeat steps 1 – 5 on the other side.

7. Afterwards, notice the sensations in your legs, and whether you feel like your mental condition has also changed.

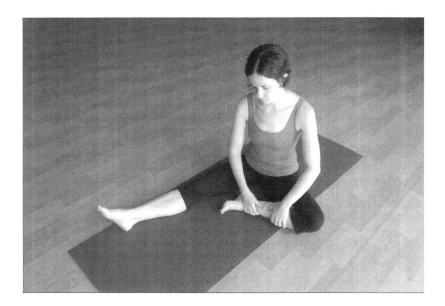

Forward Bend

1. Sit with your legs straight out in front of you.

2. Place the bolster (or a few pillows) on your thighs. Be sure not to cramp your belly area; give it some space.

3. When you're ready, simply inhale, draw the arms above the head, and get some length on the spine. Then as you exhale, draw your chest forward and down over the legs. You don't have to be able to grab your feet—that's not important. Your hands go anywhere that is comfortable; on the floor, on your legs, or on your feet is fine.

4. Take your time and be patient. It takes a while for some tissues in the body to respond, so just keep breathing and keep softening into it. We want to get to a point where gravity is doing most of the work for you; you just have to soften your body and allow it to move further down towards the floor. Relax your shoulders and arms, no need to hold on here...

5. Allow the back to curl, and relax your head to rest the forehead onto the bolster or pillows. Close the eyes, soften the body, and breathe. Hold for at least three minutes if comfortable. Feel free to come out if you feel like you've had enough. (Try not to come out until you have found at least one moment of peace within the pose.)

Variations:

1. If you are having difficulty getting your chest and torso forward, then try sitting up on some blankets or some cushions so

your hips are off the floor. This helps the upper body to be able to come forward over the legs. Experiment with the height of the hips if you need to. With this one, you are looking to find a place where gravity takes over and draws your torso down towards the legs.

2. If you have trouble getting your head to sit on the bolster or the pillows, you may need to increase the amount of pillows and cushions so that your head can find a place to rest on them. If that is too distracting or you don't have enough pillows to make it work, try not using any pillows or supports and letting your head hang in space towards the floor. Relax your neck and let gravity draw your head down. Breathe. Soften.

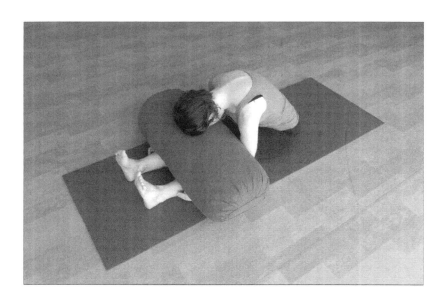

Reclining Bridge

This is one of my favorites. This is an amazing pose to release the lower back, and it sends blood and nutrients to the lungs, heart and brain.

To set yourself up for this pose, you will need a bolster or some big blocky cushions. Pillows are unlikely to be enough here. Bring the bolster or blocky cushions lengthwise down the mat, so that your hips and legs can be supported and off the floor, like in the picture above.

1. To get into position, line up the bolster, and maybe add an extra pillow, cushion, or bolster if you have long legs, like me.

2. Sit up and straddle the bolster, with legs on either side. Then start to lie back. Make sure the bolster sits nicely into the lower back supporting the sacrum. Don't let it come up so it is touching your ribs; you want it lower than that, so it sits nicely in the lower back curve. Your shoulders should easily rest on the floor or mat. You can use a folded blanket under the head if you need the extra support.

3. Bring the legs up onto the bolster. You will need to bring the legs comfortably together, and let the feet splay out to the sides.

4. Relax the arms down the side of the body and soften the back of the neck.

5. Stay for at least 3 – 5 minutes. Take your time. Close your eyes. Breathe gently.

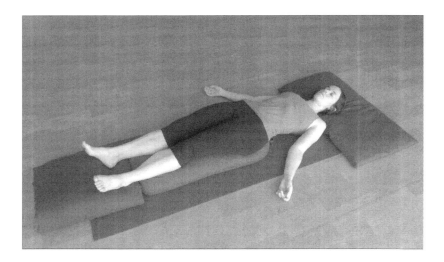

Variation:

1. Sometimes the legs won't stay up on the bolster, as they can slip off the sides. If you have this issue then, when you are straddling the bolster and ready to lie back, try strapping your legs together around the calf muscles with a yoga strap or a belt. Keep your knees bent so you can recline more easily. When your back is settled on the floor, extend the legs out on top of the bolster. Then recline down towards the mat, and when your back is settled, bring the legs up to rest on the bolster. Let the feet splay out to the sides. The strap should hold the legs together so you can really let go of the legs.

The Hug

1. Come to sit upright on the heels, with the tops of the feet flat.

2. Spread your knees apart so they are comfortable.

3. Bring the bolster and/or pillows in between the legs. Be sure not to jam the bolster and pillows into your belly; give your belly some space so it can relax and not be cramped up. You can add a little cushion or pillow just for your head if that feels good.

4. When you're ready, just bring the torso forward and down over the bolster and pillows. Rest your head to one side.

5. I find bringing the arms up to hug the bolster gives a nice release for the upper back.

6. Rest and relax; breathe gently.

7. Be sure to rest your head in the other direction at some point.

8. You can stay for at least three minutes in this one. Continue to breathe gently. Close the eyes. Feel the whole of the back gently open and soften.

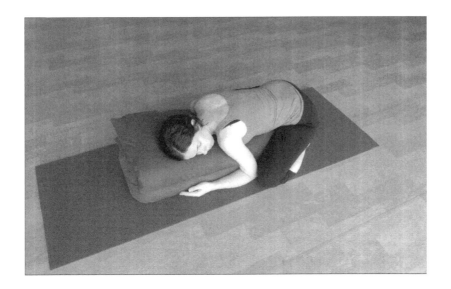

Variations:

1. If your knees don't feel good when sitting this way, you can bring a few blankets between your heels and your buttocks or hamstrings. This will take the pressure off of the knees.

2. If your ankles or feet don't feel good when sitting this way, try bringing a rolled up blanket or small cushion under the front of your ankles, so that the foot and ankle will have more of a natural angle and not be so flat against the floor. Feel free to experiment to find a position that works for you. When you bring your weight forward over the bolsters and pillows, it will take a lot of the weight off of the feet also.

3. If you have trouble bringing the torso down to rest on the bolster and pillow supports, then you may just need to bulk up your support with more pillows, blankets and bolsters, so that you can rest the head and torso. Again, feel free to experiment.

The Hug with a Twist

This is a variation of the hug, and can be done after the hug or on its own—but be sure to do both sides. This pose allows for the most amazing opening, which goes diagonally across the back from the shoulder to the opposite hip.

1. To set yourself up, bring both knees over to your right side so you are sitting on your left hip.

2. Bring the bolster and pillows lengthwise, and draw them in towards your belly. Do not jam them up into your belly; allow a little space. Just make sure the knees are actually coming up beside the bolster and pillow supports. Again, feel free to add a little cushion for the head if that feels good.

3. When you are ready, bring the torso forward and down so that the chest comes to rest onto the bolster and pillows. At first, rest the head in the direction of the knees; after a while you can change the head to the other direction if it feels good for your neck.

4. Allow the body to soften. You can bring your hands up and hug the bolster and pillows.

5. Relax your shoulders. Relax your back. Breathe easily. You can stay here for around 2 – 3 minutes.

6. Finally, when you're ready, draw yourself up, slowly swap your legs over to the other side, and repeat.

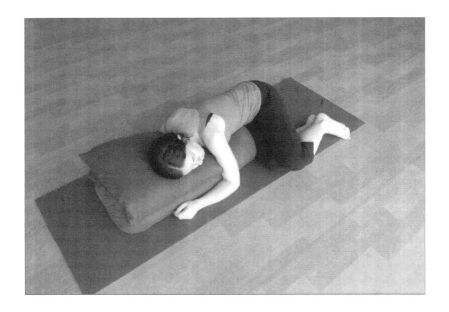

Supported Hips Pose

1. Sit up naturally on your mat and bring the bolster crosswise into the middle of your mat.

2. Sit on top of the bolster with your knees bent.

3. When you're ready, slowly lower your back and torso towards the floor, using your arms for support. (There is another way to get into this position, which I have explained in the "Variations" section that comes next.)

4. Make sure your shoulders rest comfortably on the floor. Also, make sure that the bolster is comfortably in your lower back curve; don't let it come up to touch the lower ribs.

5. Make sure your sacrum and your hips sit comfortably on the bolster.

6. You can bring a folded blanket under the back of your head if you wish.

7. You can keep your knees bent, or, some people like to extend the legs out straight. Do whatever feels good for you.

8. Stay here as long as comfortable, at least 2 – 3 minutes.

Variation:

1. Another way to get into this pose that may be easier for you is to simply lie flat on your back on the floor. Then bend the knees, push the feet into the floor to raise the hips towards the sky, and

slide the bolster in underneath the sacrum and hip area. Relax the hips down onto the bolster. Adjust as necessary; check step four for correct positioning.

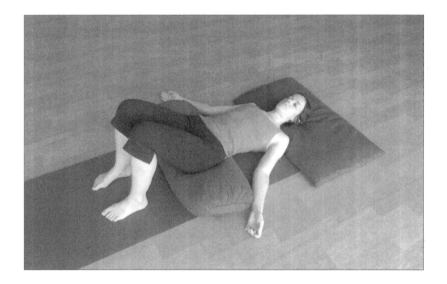

Supported Hips with a Twist

This is an extension of the previous pose (supported hips pose).

You will need extra pillows or a bolster for this one.

1. Have an extra pillow and/or bolster close by so you can move it into position after you have found your way into supported hips pose.

2. After you have gotten yourself into supported hips pose with your knees bent, find a way to bring the extra pillow or bolster just to the left side of the bolster that is already under your hips.

3. Then, when you are ready, bring your feet off the floor and your knees towards your chest, and then let the knees and legs drop gently over to the left side. Come to rest your lower legs on the extra pillow and bolster. Adjust the support so it is comfortable.

4. You should now have your hips elevated on the original bolster, and you should also have your lower legs supported over the left side so that your hips, lower back, and upper back are twisting.

5. Keep the head looking upwards, and relax the arms wherever they are comfortable.

6. We tend not to stay in this twist as long as the original supported hip pose; we usually come out after a minute or two. If you wish to stay longer you can, but don't overdo it.

7. When you've had enough, try going to the other side. Bring your knees and lower legs up over your chest. Find a way to get the extra bolster and pillow over to the right side, and when ready, lower the legs over to the right side.

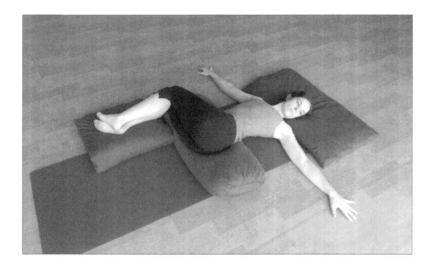

Legs Up the Wall

This is a great pose to start off with, especially if you have been on your feet all day. It drains the feet and flushes the organs with blood and nutrients. This is a safe variation for all.

1. Getting into this position can be a bit awkward. If you have a bolster available you keep it close and within arms reach. However, if you don't have a bolster, it doesn't matter because keeping your hips on the mat is good too. To start, the key is to sit up alongside a wall, getting as close as you can to the wall with one hip.

2. Then, roll yourself down onto your back and shoot your legs up the wall. Ideally the buttocks are quite close to the wall, though people who have tight hamstrings will need to come away from the wall so they can get their legs up. In this case, the knees will probably be bent, but that's okay. If your hamstrings are okay, wiggle yourself closer to the wall so your buttocks touch the wall.

3. If you want to add the bolster for extra support, then grab the bolster and bring it close to your hips. Place your feet onto the wall and push the feet into the wall so you can raise your buttocks and hips off the floor slightly. Then quickly slide the bolster under where your hips would be if they were on the floor. Then lower your hips down onto the bolster. Once you find a comfortable position, let your arms fall away to the side, close your eyes, and just relax with a gentle breath. You can stay here for 3 – 15 minutes.

4. To come out, bend the knees, then roll to your right side. Wait here for a minute or two so the legs can get some blood back into

them before moving or standing. Take your time... if the phone rings or something like this, let it go… do not rush out of this one.

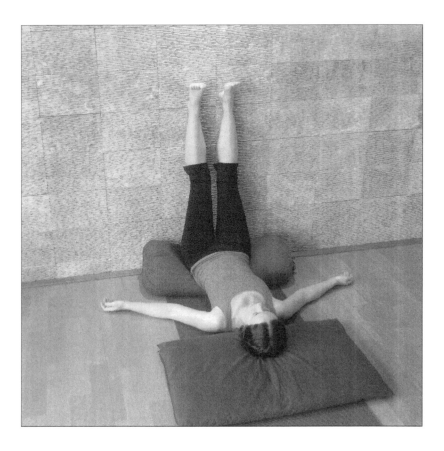

Variations:

1. If the hamstrings are tight, just wiggle yourself away from the wall until you find a comfortable position where your legs can rest against the wall. Your knees will probably be bent, but that's ok.

2. Sometimes the legs want to fall away to the sides, and it's hard to relax them because you have to hold them up there. If this

happens, you can strap your legs together with a yoga strap, a belt, or anything really. Strap them together around the calf muscle area. To do this, when you get onto your back, bend your knees into your chest, and then strap the legs together. When done, extend them up the wall and wiggle yourself into a comfortable position.

3. Simply bring the soles of the feet together and let the knees fall out to the side.

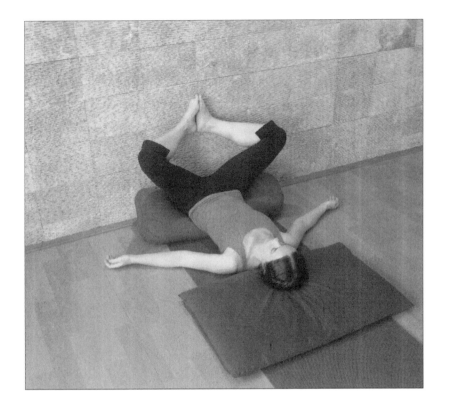

Supported Lower Back Curl

This is similar to the supported hips pose, but this time the bolster comes up higher so it's sitting right in the curve of the lower back. This is a good pose for digestion and opening the abdominal cavity.

1. To get into this position, sit up naturally on the mat and bring the bolster just behind your hips so that the bolster sits crosswise on the mat.

2. Now, bend the knees and start to lower your upper back to the floor, allowing the lower back to fully curl over the bolster. The bolster will be touching your lower ribs. For some people the buttocks rest on the floor, but for others the buttocks may be slightly off the floor. As long as there is no muscular effort involved, it is fine either way. Do whatever feels more natural for you.

Please note: For some people the bolster feels too big. If this is the case for you, you can use a folded up pillow instead, or a smaller bolster if you have one, and try getting into the pose again. Find a position that is comfortable.

3. Relax the arms wherever is comfortable. You might like to bring the arms up overhead for a further opening in the front of the body.

4. You can keep the knees bent or bring them straight, whatever feels better for you. Relax the head into a natural position.

5. Breathe gently and stay for at least three minutes.

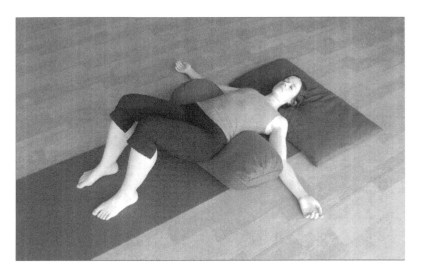

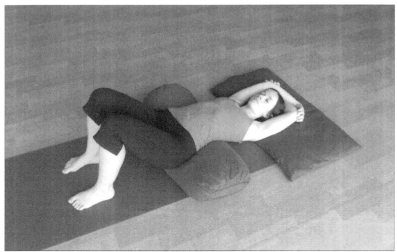

Natural Twist

This pose usually requires no support or props, though some people benefit from having something under the bent leg. Try it without the support first, but if it feels too strenuous or your breath is halted, then you may need to use a bolster or pillow under the bent leg. Have a bolster or pillow nearby just in case.

1. To get into this position, first just lay flat out onto the floor.

2. Bring the left arm out to the side at about shoulder height, keeping your elbow bent or your arm straight; whichever feels better and whatever you have the space for.

3. Bend your left knee so that the knee joint is sitting comfortably at about ninety degrees.

4. Bring your right hand to your left knee and start to guide the knee across your body so that you come into a twist.

5. Let the leg come as far over towards the floor as possible. It you start straining, then wither back off a bit, or bring a bolster or pillow under that bent leg so it can come to relax.

6. Find a comfortable position in which you can breathe smoothly.

7. If your neck is okay, try looking back over your left arm.

8. Stay for at least one minute.

9. Release by bringing the bent leg back up to the middle and straightening out both legs. Rest for a moment, then go to the other side.

10. Repeat steps 2 – 8 with the opposite arms and legs.

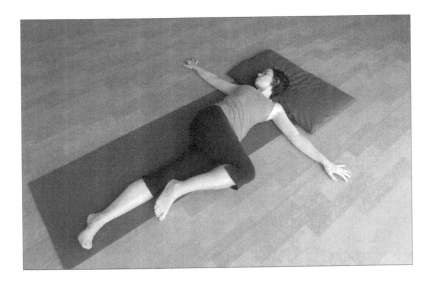

Release for the Back

This little exercise is great for releasing small groups of vertebrae up and down the spine. I have had a number of chiropractors and physiotherapists recommend this as a way to release the spine and the back muscles.

1. First, grab a spare yoga mat or a bath towel and roll it up like in the picture below.

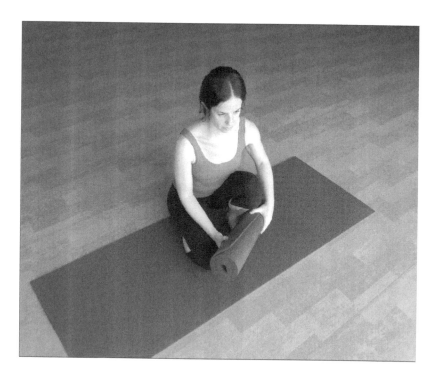

2. Then start by bringing it crosswise into your lower back. You can either slide it under your back when lying down, or you can

sit up first and the lie down over the mat or towel. Do whichever feels better for you.

3. Make sure the mat or towel is at a straight angle across the back; avoid diagonals.

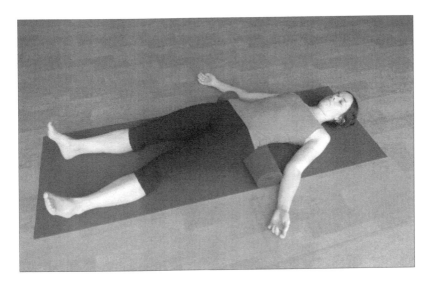

4. Stay for about 2 – 3 minutes, but no longer than five minutes—and please don't fall asleep like this! It can cause some problems if you fall asleep in this position for a long time.

5. Start to adjust the mat or towel so it moves up the spine, moving only a few inches at a time. You can adjust it by bending the knees and raising the hips up, and then sliding the towel up underneath you, or you can sit up, move the towel and then lie back down. You choose.

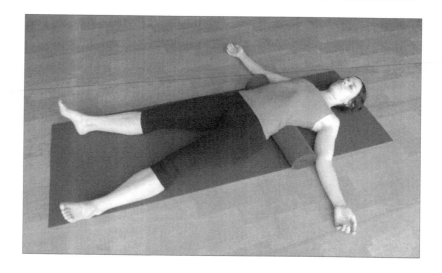

6. Again, only stay for a maximum of about five minutes, and then adjust the mat or towel again, going higher up the spine a few inches.

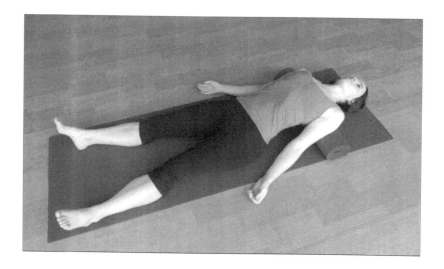

7. Repeat the process until you reach the back of the neck. Repeat with the neck; allow the neck to find its curve over the mat or towel.

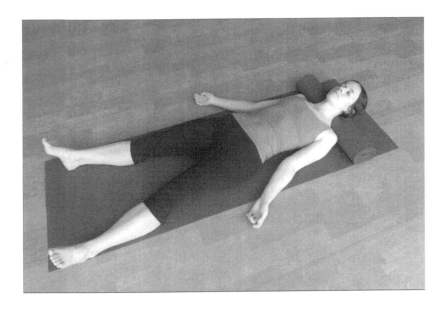

8. After a few minutes, release and sit up for the next pose, or just come into final relaxation pose - Shavasana.

Shavasana (Corpse Pose)
Final relaxation pose

This is the pose you always need to finish any sequence with. The body needs a moment to settle and reorganize itself. It is very powerful and should not be skipped over. Even just one minute can bring much benefit. There are many variations to this pose, but one thing remains consistent – the total relaxation of the body in the supine position.

1. Lie straight out on the floor with your legs extended.

2. Place legs slightly apart, with feet splaying out to the sides.

3. Your arms should lie just away from the body, with palms facing up or down. Or, you can place your palms onto your chest or belly, which ever feels right for you.

4. Close your eyes. Relax the eyes into the sockets.

5. Have a quick scan through your body, moving your awareness through your feet, legs, hips, back, belly, chest, arms, shoulders, neck and head. Check to make sure that you're not holding on to any tension in the body.

6. Stay for 1 – 5 minutes. Try not to move your body; just remain still. Relinquish thoughts as they arise; don't give them any importance, just let them go for now.

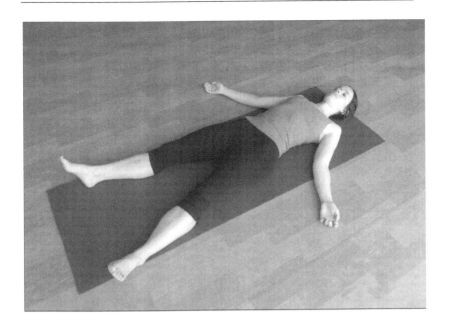

Variations:

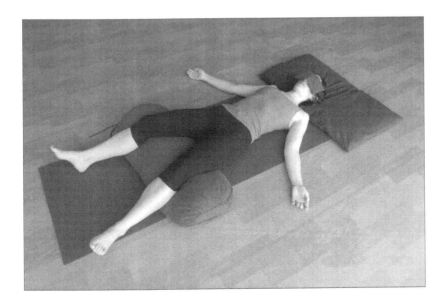

1. You might like to try bringing a bolster or pillow supports under the knees. This helps soften the lower back towards the floor. Therefore, this is <u>recommended if you have lower back pain</u> or problems. Also, if you have an eye pillow, now is a good time to use it. Something placed under the back of head to raise the head slightly off the floor can help relax the muscles in the neck. However, avoid big fluffy pillows because they can raise the head to high and create strain in the neck.

2. Follow steps 3 – 6.

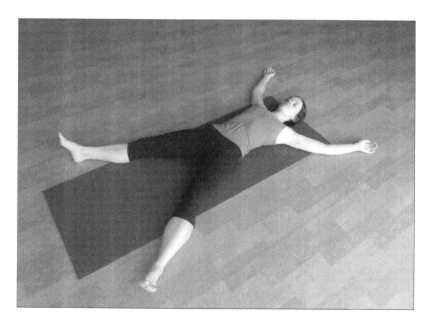

1. Find a comfortable position by bringing the arms out diagonally above the head and widen the legs slightly.

2. Close your eyes and let your body completely rest for at least 1-5 minutes.

Practice Sequences

*'Besides the noble art of getting things done, there is
The nobler art of leaving things undone."*

~ Lin Yutang

This chapter of the book focuses on specific sequences using restorative yoga poses. Over time, as you become more familiar with the poses, feel free to adjust the sequences to suit you. They have been divided into different categories. They are:

10 minutes

20 minutes

30 minutes

60 minutes or more...

Lower Back Pain Poses

Women's Health

Tight Hips

10 minutes—Need to Chill Out ASAP!

Massage the Legs

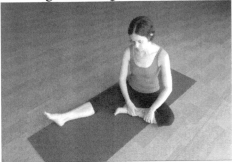

Supported Butterfly

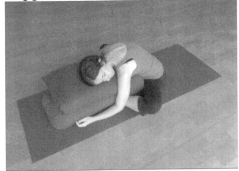

Reclining Bridge

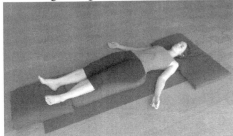

Shavasana

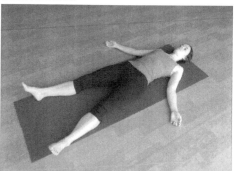

20 minutes

Supported Butterfly

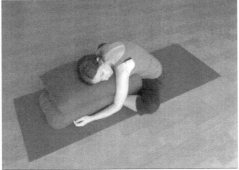

Massage the Legs

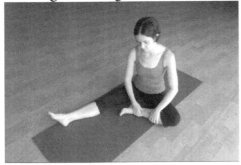

Forward Bend

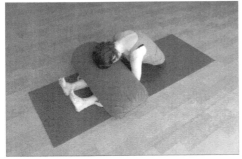

Supported Hips

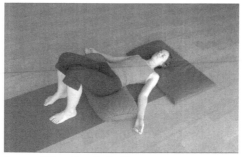

Legs Up the Wall

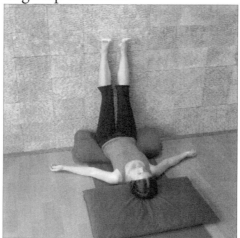

Rest / Shavasana

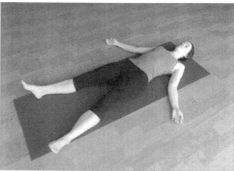

30 minutes

Supported Butterfly

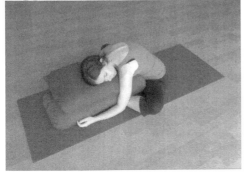

Massage the Legs

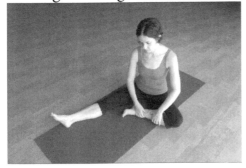

Supported Hips

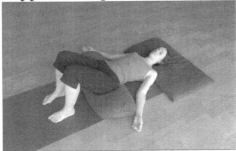

Supported Hips Twist

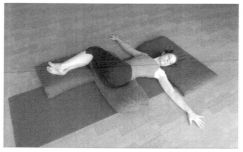

The Hug

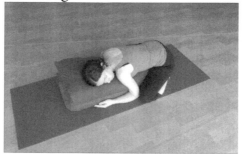

The Hug with a Twist

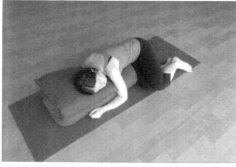

Rest / Shavasana

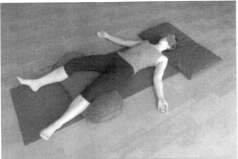

60 minutes or more...

Butterfly

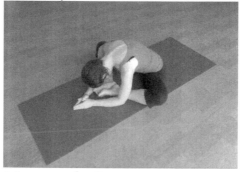

Massage the Legs

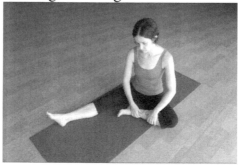

Supported Forward Bend

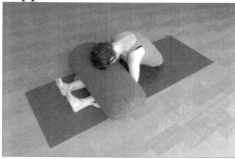

Reclining Bridge

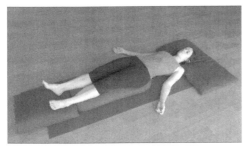

The Hug

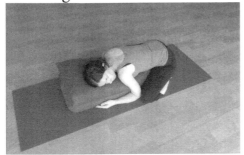

The Hug with a Twist

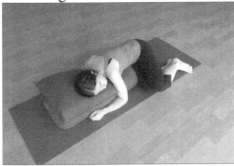

Supported Hips

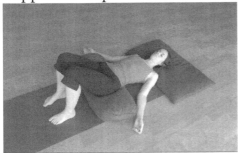

Legs Up the Wall

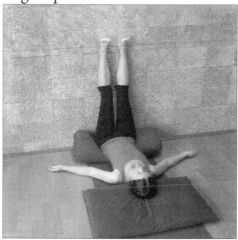

Towel Release for the Back

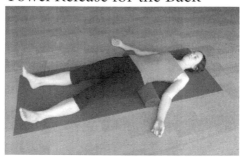

Natural Twist

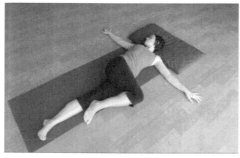

Rest / Shavasana

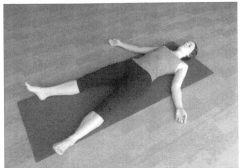

Lower Back Pain Poses

Butterfly

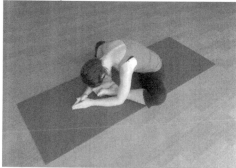

Forward Bend

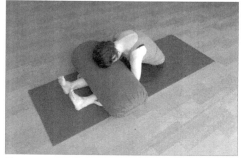

Supported Hips

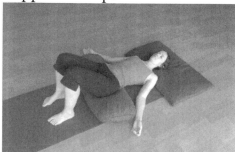

Supported Hip Twist

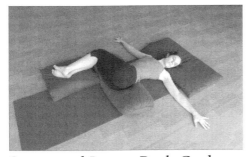

Supported Lower Back Curl

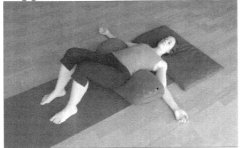

The Hug

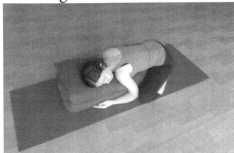

The Hug with a Twist

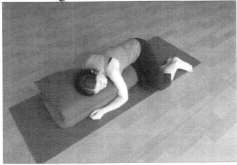

Natural Twist

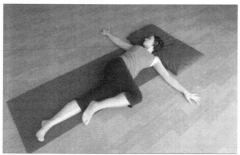

Rest / Shavasana

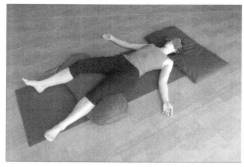

Women's Health

Butterfly

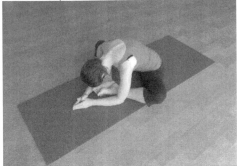

The Hug

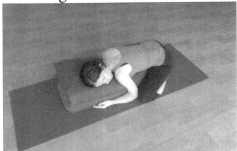

The Hug with a Twist

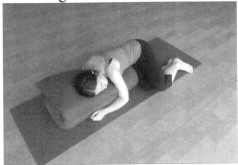

Supported Hips Pose

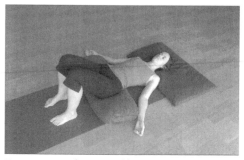

Legs Up the Wall

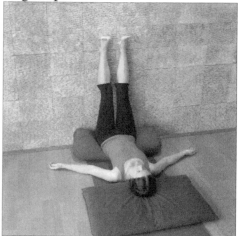

Forward Bend

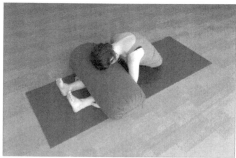

Rest / Shavasana

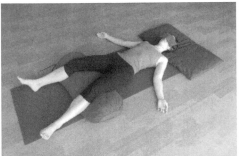

Tight Hips

Massage the Legs

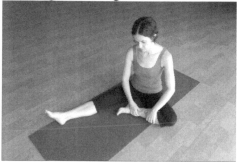

Supported Butterfly

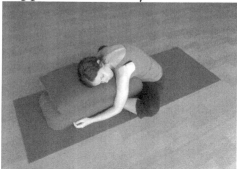

The Hug

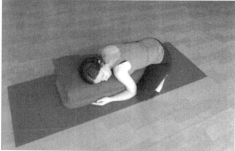

The Hug with a Twist

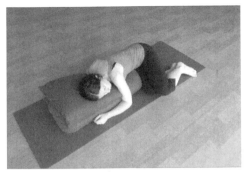

Forward Bend

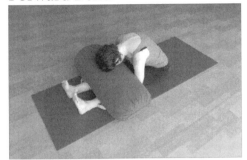

Rest / Shavasana

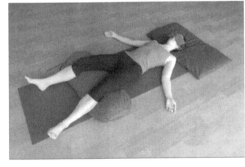

Meditation and Mindfulness Practices

Restorative yoga is not only about placing the body into restful poses; it is also about resting the mind and all the associated mental activity. The mind has a tendency to play out into past memories, future 'what if' scenarios and into imagination whenever it gets the chance. Therefore, as with the body, the mental energies of the mind also require periods of rest or de-energizing. There are a variety of methods and techniques one can employ to initiate change in the behavior of the mind and this chapter is dedicated to discussing some of the simplest and most effective methods. Many people believe that the mind needs to be stopped from its thinking. The mind is designed to think and it will continue to think whether you want it to stop or not. It's a matter of attention. The more attention you give the mind and its thoughts, the louder and more consuming they appear. A better approach is to allow the mind to think but place your attention away from this mental activity. Instead, focus your attention on your breath, the sensations in your body, the space in-between the thoughts or onto the one who is witnessing the thoughts occurring.

The following chapter explores, in more detail, various techniques to help de-emphasize and essentially de-energize the activity of the mind and place your attention elsewhere.

Breath Awareness (Breath Attention)

One of the most effective methods is through the breath. The breath provides us with a simple anchor that draws us into the present moment of our experience. Simply place your attention on your breath as it travels in and out of the nostrils. Modern day humans also have a tendency to over breathe, to breathe too rapidly as well as to not breathe out enough. If we revisit the theory of yin and yang, yang relates to breathing in and yin is breathing out and letting go. If we breathe in more than we breathe out, we are encouraging more yang activity in our systems. Therefore, we can easily alter this yang dominant pattern of breath by simply taking some time to use extended exhales.

1. Get yourself into your physical pose (posture) and, when you're ready, close your eyes.

2. Draw your attention to your breath and notice how you're breathing. Do not try to alter or change it at this stage, just become aware of yourself breathing for a few minutes.

3. After a few minutes, start to alter the breath slightly by slowing your breathing down. Increase both your inhales and your exhales in a gentle way. Do not force or strain yourself.

4. After a few minutes of slightly deepened breathing, now make your exhale breath slightly longer than your inhale breath. You can add a count to the breath if that helps with your focus and your connection to your breath e.g. 4 beats inhale and 6 beats exhale. If the counting doesn't work for you, that's ok, you don't have to use it. With your awareness you should be able to sense, by listening to your breath, if your exhale is slightly longer than your inhale. If you can sense this, then just keep to that practice and let any thoughts pass. Keep the breath moving and flowing, like waves bobbing on the ocean.

Bodily Sensations Awareness

Another technique is to cycle your awareness to various points throughout your body. This is a very powerful technique that helps to re-connect the mind to the body. Giving your mind a task will also keep it occupied and, if you place the mind's attention into your body sensation, you can more effectively relax the body and eventually enhance your ability to sense more subtle energetics.

1. Start by drawing your attention down onto your feet. Sense the soles of the feet, the top of the foot and then the ankle.

2. Start to move your awareness up your body, part by part. Sense the calves, the knees, the thighs to the hips.

3. Sense the lower back, the upper back, the left shoulder and the right shoulder.

4. Sense the left side of the chest, the right side of the chest, the upper belly and the lower belly.

5. Then travel your awareness down one arm to the fingers and then move down the other arm to the fingers.

6. Become aware of your neck, jaw, cheeks, forehead and the top of your head.

Then allow yourself to feel the whole body all at once. Can you sense it? If not, do another scan. Start at the feet and work your way up. Each time you scan your body you will be able to sense it much easier and the sense will remain for longer periods, even after the practice.

It is not absolutely necessary that you move in this way, from feet to head. You can change the way you move the awareness through the body, however it is advisable to stay with the same pattern of movement once you have established your process. After a few scans in one direction, try moving in the other direction also, e.g. from head to feet.

Chakra Meditation

Another technique is to focus your attention on the chakras, one at a time, and use your breath and an internal mantra to balance and emphasize the energy center. There are 7 primary chakras that are located along the spine, starting from the base of the torso up to the crown of the head. If you are unfamiliar with them or want to know more about them there are hundreds of books out there that go into great detail if you want to learn more about the chakras. Working with the chakras is specifically good for healing the physical and balancing out the emotional and mental energies.

1. Begin by getting yourself set up into any restorative yoga pose.

2. Once you are comfortable, start by placing your attention at the base chakra (Base of Torso, around the genital area) and allow the space to relax if you find yourself holding any tension in the area.

3. Place the tongue on the tip of the top of the mouth and allow yourself to breathe steadily and easily through the nose.

3. Keeping your attention on the base chakra area as you breathe in, internally chant to yourself "Sooooo" and, as you breathe out, chant internally to yourself "Huummmmm".

4. Continue a few breathes in this way. Be sure not to strain with this, it can be easy to "try to hard". Find an easy and relaxed way of doing it. You will find an easy way to do it after a few minutes of practice.

5. After around 10 breaths, move your awareness up to the next chakra (The Sacral—just below the belly button). Again repeat the process. As you breathe in, internally chant "Sooooo," and, as you breathe out, internally chant "Hummmmm".

6. After around 10 breaths, move your awareness up to the next chakra (The Solar Plexus—upper abdomen). Again repeat the process. As you breathe in, internally chant "Sooooo," and, as you breathe out, internally chant "Hummmmm".

7. After around 10 breaths, move your awareness up to the next chakra (The Heart—centre of chest). Again repeat the process. As you breathe in, internally chant "Sooooo," and, as you breathe out, internally chant "Hummmmm".

8. After around 10 breaths, move your awareness up to the next chakra (The Throat—base of the throat). Again repeat the process. As you breathe in, internally chant "Sooooo," and, as you breathe out, internally chant "Hummmmm".

9. After around 10 breaths, move your awareness up to the next chakra (The Third Eye—middle of the eyebrows). Again repeat the process. As you breathe in, internally chant "Sooooo," and, as you breathe out, internally chant "Hummmmm".

10. After around 10 breaths, move your awareness up to the next chakra (The Crown—top of the head). Again repeat the process. As you breathe in, internally chant "Sooooo," and, as you breathe out, internally chant "Hummmmm".

This technique can be used in a variety of circumstances and is therefore not limited to a restorative yoga practice. For example, this technique is very suitable for those who may have become sick and are bedridden. Working with the chakras in this way can greatly reduce their suffering and enhance recovery.

Mastering Emotions

What inevitably occurs, when we slow down and rest in silence, is that suppressed emotions and feelings will rise to the surface. Most of us are taught either to run away from them, distract ourselves, suppress them, express them, pop a pill or seek another more pleasant emotion or experience in order to deal with and manage uncomfortable emotions and feelings. When we do this, we are resisting. When we resist, it will persist. When we don't allow the time and the space for the uncomfortable feelings and emotions to run their course and dissipate, they become suppressed, energized and will arise again in the near future.

Restorative Yoga is a powerful practice, similar to that of mediation, because it actually encourages suppressed and often uncomfortable emotions and feelings to come to the surface to be dealt with and processed. The teaching here is, instead of running away from these uncomfortable feelings and emotions, try leaning into them instead. Do not resist the feelings in running their course throughout your body, watch them objectively as they arise, remain as a witness and then we won't react. Do not feed the uncomfortable feelings or follow the stories the mind comes up with in regards to the feelings. Surrender to them and go to the depths of them. Eventually, you will find they will run out of energy and intensity and they will dissipate. Along with the feelings, all associated thoughts and stories will be eliminated.

If the emotions or feelings come from a very traumatic experience, it may be better to deal with them in small chunks rather than taking on the whole thing. Just chip away at them. When it gets too much, then you can distract yourself or do whatever it is that you do but remember to return to them with openness next time and continue working with them.

When we resist good or bad feelings, we resist our humanness. Being human involves a vast range of feelings and emotions. Learning to experience the full spectrum of our feelings without reacting to them, automatically cultivates compassion for ourselves and towards other beings because we understand on the deepest level how they feel. When we learn to be ok with the full spectrum of our feelings—the good, the bad and the ugly—it builds a sense of inner confidence and of self-assurance because we know that we are able to manage any experience or feelings as they arise. We become connected, grounded and fully present to our feelings, sensations and experiences when we fully accept them and don't resist them.

So, when you are next practicing restorative yoga and you are met inside with an uncomfortable emotional feeling, become the witness to it and try leaning into it instead of running away and see for yourself.

"There are times when we stop. We sit still... we listen and breezes from a whole other world begin to appear."

~ James Carroll

Resources

Yoga Supplies

USA:
www.manduka.com

www.gaiam.com

www.barefootyoga.com

UK:
www.yogamatters.com

www.yogamad.com

Australia:
www.iyogaprops.com.au

www.empind.com.au

Yoga Music

www.soundstrue.com

www.yogi-tunes.com

Yoga Classes Online

www.myyogaonline.com.au

A Little Bit About The Author

When I was younger I played a lot of sports at school. Not very well, but I tried my best. After I left school I pretty much quit all of my sporting activities and drifted for many years, avoiding university and any serious commitment to a working life or career. This was a blessing, as it gave me time and space to explore the world around me and see what was out there.

I traveled around Australia and New Zealand, and ended up in China teaching English for a year. When I returned, I started studying remedial massage and Chinese medicine at a community health college close to my house. Before I went traveling, I had started training in Capoeira while living near Sydney. Capoeira is a Brazilian martial art that is very dynamic and acrobatic, being described as more of a dance than a martial art. I trained in Capoeira for four good years and really loved it, but found it very competitive.

It was during the last years of my Capoeira training that I began exploring various types of yoga practices in my home town. I was looking for benefits similar to those that Capoeira provided, but with less ego, and more of a philosophical and spiritual context. It was in 2002 that I discovered a gentle yoga style known as Oki-Do yoga in Brisbane, Australia. Oki-Do yoga comes from a Japanese Zen master teacher known as Dr. Masahiro Oki. The Oki-Do style is very nurturing, as it incorporates many shiatsu and massage techniques, yet it can also be very energizing and stimulating when working with *hara* (lower belly) training and asana practices.

From that point on I was pretty much hooked on yoga, and gave up Capoeira. In 2009 I underwent my teacher training in traditional Indian hatha yoga, as I was wanting to deepen my understanding of Indian yoga and philosophy. At this same time I was also completing my formal studies in acupuncture and Chinese medicine. It was through my formal education as well as my practice with various yoga forms that I came to see the importance of having a gentle practice alongside a more vigorous and energetic practice. There was also an obvious link to the seasons and the time of day as to which practice is more suitable. For example, yang rises in the morning, so stronger practices are better in the morning, and yin falls in the evening, so more gentle and creative pursuits are better at night.

I began teaching yoga soon after I completed my teacher training. I taught mainly hatha, vinyasa flow, and some Qi Gong when I started out. These days, everywhere I look the yoga world is full of the "hot" and "power", "yang" yoga styles of practice. While these practices are required and necessary, there seems to be a real lack of "yin" yoga practices available to the modern yoga enthusiast.

For this reason, in the last few years I have really been focusing on teaching "yin" style yoga forms, like restorative, gentle, beginners', yin yoga, yoga nidra, and Buddhist and yogic meditation in studios. I am pleased to say that no matter when I go, the local community always warmly welcomes these practices. To further promote, encourage and cultivate the practice of "yin" style yoga, I have written this book. I hope you have gained a deeper understanding from this book, and I also hope you feel confident enough to start incorporating some of these techniques into your yoga practice.

Namaste

"Muddy water, let stand, becomes clear."

~ Lao Tzu

Other Books By This Author

www.michaelhetherington.com.au

www.amazon.com

Chakra Balancing Made Simple and Easy

The Complete Book of Oriental Yoga

Meditation Made Simple

The Little Book of Yin

How to Learn Acupuncture

Simply Zen Quotes

Made in the USA
San Bernardino, CA
11 July 2014